Home
Spinal
Care

Contents

Legal Notice
and Disclaimer

The Problem

Did you know that your spine should be in a certain alignment? Did you know it should move through a full range of motion in each direction, and it should be free of aches and pains? These are the most basic facts when it comes to spinal care and our society for the most part doesn't have a clue.

If you skip to the last chapter of this book you will find all the home spinal care procedures you are looking for and exactly how to perform them safely. That being said, I highly recommend you do NOT skip to the end! This entire book is important. If you really want to build a healthy spine I suggest you read it all.

In these next several chapters we will discuss why there are so many spinal health problems in our society, what causes spinal problems, and how to correct them once and for all.

If you are reading this and you don't have a spinal problem, that's great. This book will help you understand how and why you should continue to maintain the health of your spine. If you do have a spinal problem that is great too (well, that's not great, but you know what I mean...). This book will help you understand what your problem might be, what might have caused it and where you can go from here.

Most of us understand that every part of our body needs to be taken care of. We see the dentist regularly to maintain oral hygiene. We schedule physicals, mammograms, and colonoscopies as regular wellness checkups. You are taught from a very young age that you must brush your teeth a couple times a day and floss at least once a day if you want to have a healthy smile. Basically, we are taught that if we don't do proper upkeep on all areas of our body it won't last as long as we want it to.

That said, spinal health seems to fly under the radar in our society. No one is taught to take care of their spine. If you ask anyone what spinal hygiene is, or how to properly take care of your spine there is a very good chance all you will get is a funny stare!

I am a Chiropractor and I work with the spine all day long, every day. I have seen literally thousands of spinal x-rays. I have seen x-rays of 4 year olds , 94 year olds, and everything in-between. Most of the pictures I see are not pretty at all. This is because no one knows how to properly maintain the health of their spine.

If you will allow me, I would like to show you exactly what I am talking about. Just like your teeth your spine was meant to be in a certain alignment. If you study every text book ever made about health, check out every anatomy book at your local library, and scavenge every book used in any medical school in the world, they will all tell you the same thing – The spine should be in a certain alignment!

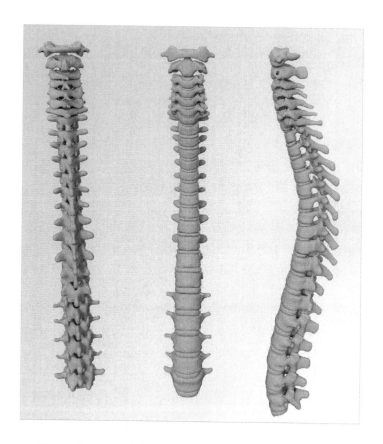

The spine should be straight from front to back and from the side it shouldn't be straight. Looking at it from the side we should see 3 curves – one in the neck, one in the upper back, and one in the lower back. The curve in the neck is very important to keep the head over the shoulders and it is called a lordosis. The curve in the upper back is the opposite direction and is called a kyphosis. The curve in the low back goes the same direction as the one in the neck and is also called a lordosis.

Whether you are 2 or 102 (years of age) your spine should have this proper alignment!

Your spine has 24 movable bones we call vertebrae.

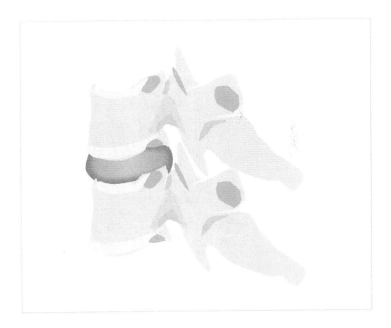

Each one should move through a full range of motion. The spine should be able to flex all the way forward as you touch your toes and then bend backwards as you look up at the ceiling. It should bend sideways to both sides and it should also rotate fully to both sides. A lot of people haven't moved their spines through a full range of motion in years.

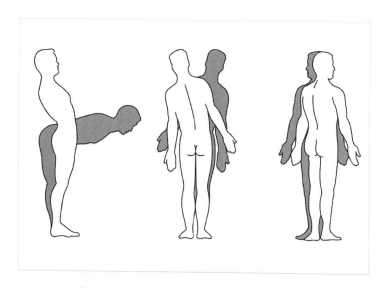

The spine should be surrounded with many strong muscles and ligaments. If any of those muscles or ligaments become weak it can make the spine more susceptible to injury and illness.

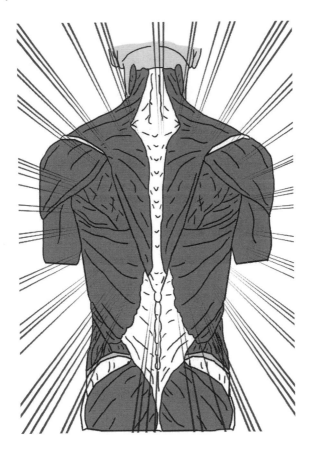

Just like the teeth, the spine will degenerate and rot if it is not properly cared for.

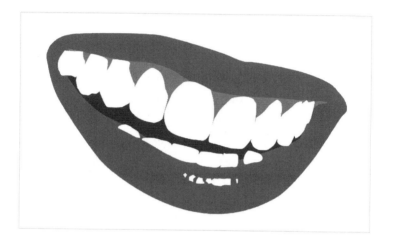

We have probably all seen the teeth of someone who has not been practicing proper oral hygiene.

But what does a spine look like if someone has not been practicing proper spinal hygiene? Spinal Degeneration is labeled in phases – Normal, Phase I, Phase II, Phase III, and sometimes even Phase IV.

We can't see spinal degeneration from looking at someone directly, but you can see it on an x-ray. The following x-rays of the neck are taken from the side.

Here is an illustration to help you understand what you are looking at:

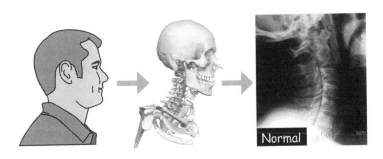

Normal

X-rays of Spinal Degeneration – Phase I-IV Below

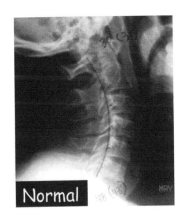

Normal

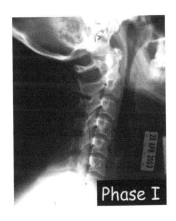

Phase I

(Loss of Curve)

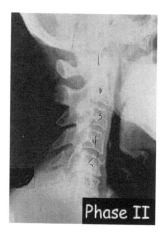

(Loss of Curve and
Degeneration)

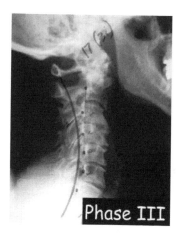

(Loss of Curve, Degeneration,
and Beginning of Fusion)

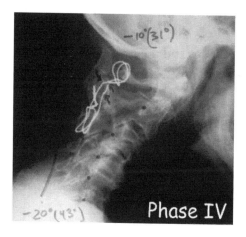

(Negative Loss of curve, Degeneration, Fusion,
and Wire in Neck from Surgery)

Can you see why it is so important to practice good spinal hygiene?

We all understand that it is very important to practice good oral hygiene, but most people don't understand that it is even more important to practice good spinal hygiene.

Just as the teeth and every other part of our body have a purpose, the spine has a very important purpose as well. It is easy to see that the purpose of the teeth is to help us chew our food. Teeth are the beginning part of the digestive process that starts every time we eat.

The purpose of the spine is to house and protect a very important organ, called the nervous system. The nervous system is a system that consists of the brain, spinal cord and nerves. It is commonly referred to as the master system of the body because it controls every function of the body, every sensation coming in or out of the body, and even your very own consciousness. To put it simply "You are your nervous system!". The spinal cord is the part of the nervous system that lies within the spine.

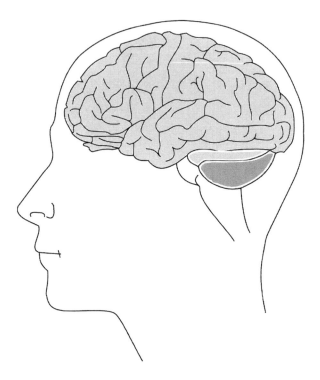

The brain constantly sends important "messages" to all 100 trillion cells in your body, coordinating each one in perfect harmony. It sends these "messages" through your spinal cord and out the nerves at each level to your organs, cells, and tissues. When the spine is unhealthy, damaged, misaligned, or stressed those messages can be affected and therefore organs, cells, and tissues can be affected.

I think Answers.com gives a great explanation of the nervous system, it says:

The main function of the Nervous System is to maintain the entire body and to also connect all your nerves; so basically, it maintains everything you do in your everyday life. Your Nervous System controls all feelings, physical or mental, such as pleasure, anger, pain, sadness, and everything else you have ever felt. Also, the brain (which is part of the nervous system) controls everything that your body should or shouldn't do. Let's think about it; do you have to think about breathing, blinking or making your heart beat? You may say no, but actually, the answer is YES! Your brain has a special part to control the things you think you don't have to think about, but are actually thinking about, all the time! So, without the brain, your lungs wouldn't breathe, you couldn't think, your heart wouldn't beat - basically you wouldn't be alive! So, you could never live without the Nervous System! (1)

The American Chiropractic Association says this about Chiropractic and the nervous system:

> Chiropractic is a health care profession that focuses on disorders of the musculoskeletal system and the nervous system, and the effects of these disorders on general health. Chiropractic care is used most often to treat neuro-musculoskeletal complaints, including but not limited to back pain, neck pain, pain in the joints of the arms or legs, and headaches.

> Doctors of Chiropractic – often referred to as chiropractors or chiropractic physicians – practice a drug-free, hands-on approach to health care that includes patient examination, diagnosis and treatment. Chiropractors have broad diagnostic skills and are also trained to recommend therapeutic and rehabilitative exercises, as well as to provide nutritional, dietary and lifestyle counseling. (2)

Now can you see why it is so important to practice good spinal hygiene?

2

Dispelling the Myths

When it comes to taking proper care of the spine have you ever said or heard someone say any of these statements before? 1) "I'm not in pain. Why should I do anything at all?" 2) "Pain and arthritis are caused from old age." 3) "It's all about genetics. My Dad had back problems and his Dad had back problems. Therefore, I am going to have back problems." Or even 4) "It is too late for me. "They" said there was nothing I could do".

Stick with me because I am about to dispel each one to those crazy myths one by one!

The first common myth is...

"I'm not in pain. Why should I do anything at all?"

What if I asked you this question, "I don't have any cavities so why should I brush my teeth?"

You would probably look at me like I lost my marbles, right?

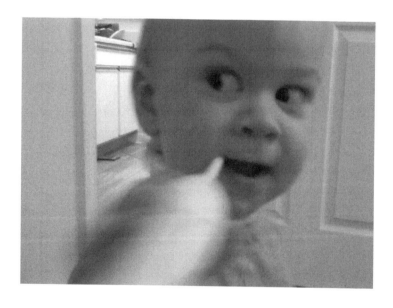

Waiting to get back pain before you start spinal care is like waiting to get a cavity before you start brushing. Once you get a cavity it's a little late.

If you are not in any pain right now, good for you! But you are exactly the one who should be reading this book. The reason we practice proper spinal hygiene is so that our spine will stay healthy (therefore keeping our body healthy). As I have said before, the spine houses the nervous system; the nervous system controls the body. So if you would like to have a long healthy life you might want to start taking care of your spine. When you are NOT in pain is the best time to start practicing spinal care.

The second common myth is...

"Pain and arthritis are caused from old age."

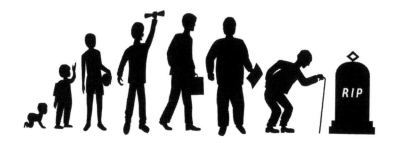

Growing old is not a disease. It shouldn't be painful or difficult. In fact, growing old should be a very pleasurable experience for everyone. Your spine should be healthy and strong no matter how old you are. I have seen people who are 80 years old and have beautiful spines. On the contrary, I have seen 26 year olds who where in terrible shape and already developing stage II degeneration in their spine.

\One of the reasons it sometimes seems that our pains get worse as we age is because of the fact that problems, in general, can get worse with time if they are not properly taken care of. This does not mean problems come with age! It means they get worse with age when not corrected.

Here are a series of x-rays taken from one person between the years of 1963 and 1975. Watch as the degeneration/arthritis continues to get worse with age (time).

"Pain and arthritis are caused from old age."

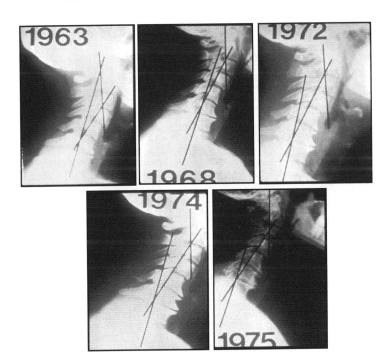

(Cervical Spine)

In the following series of x-rays you will see a before and after picture of people who got there spine corrected by a corrective care chiropractor - notice how it got better with age (time).

<u>Better with time</u>

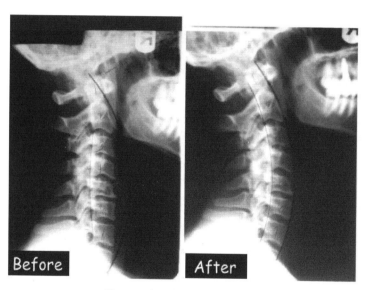

(Cervical Spine – Side view)

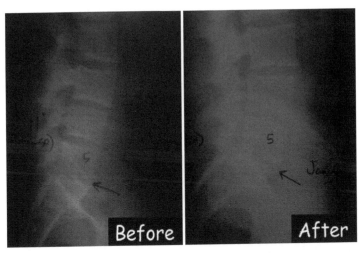

Before   After

(Lumbar Spine – Side view)

- Notice in the above x-rays, the very bottom disc space (L5) has regenerated itself (this takes a lot of work, but can be possible if proper range of motion, alignment, and overall joint integrity is restored for a long enough period of time.

A very well known medical text book called Managing Low Back Pain by Kirkaldy-Willis states that **"Aging and degenerative changes are NOT synonymous, and degenerative changes do NOT appear unless the joint has been damaged".** (3)

In the following cervical x-ray you can see that the vertebrae in the upper part of the neck (C1-C3) are healthy and show no sign of degeneration, while the vertebrae in the lower part of the neck (C5-C7) are riddled with degeneration and arthritis. If you think arthritis is caused by old age - how can some vertebrae have arthritis and some not when they are in the same spine? They can't, they are the same age. If arthritis was caused by age there would be arthritis in all the joints of the spine. Degeneration and arthritis are not caused by age, but are caused by a dysfunction in the joint and can get worse over time if not corrected.

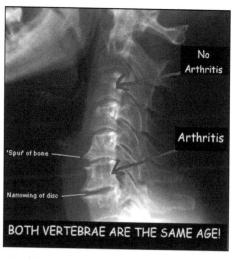

(Cervical Spine – Side view – Facing to the left)

Just like teeth, our spine can last our entire life, if we take care of it. There are many 80 year olds who have a mouth full of their own teeth. Likewise, there are many 80 year olds who have no teeth at all. Those people have to wear dentures.

The big difference between teeth and the spine is that you can get artificial teeth (they are called dentures), but you can't get an artificial spine! That is another reason it is so important to start taking care of your spine now. It doesn't matter if you are young, old, or somewhere in the middle, the best time to start taking care of your spine is today. With time and the proper care you can strengthen and build your spine no matter how old you are!

The third common myth is...

"It is all about genetics. My Dad had back problems and his Dad had back problems. Therefore, I am going to have back problems."

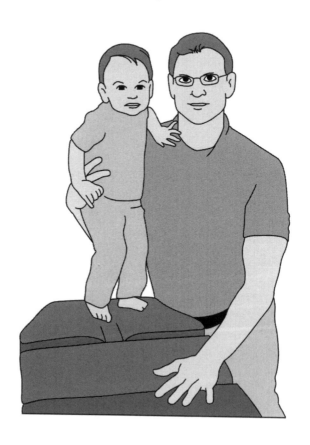

This may be the biggest myth of them all. Current science has proved that you are not slave to your genes. The idea that "You are what your genes say you are and that's final." originates with the work of Charles Darwin. Science has come a long way since then.

In Bruce Lipton's book *The Biology of Belief,* he states:

"In his 1859 book The origin of Species, Darwin said that individual traits are passed from parents to their children. He suggested that "hereditary factors" passed from parent to child control the characteristics of an individual's life. That bit of insight set scientists off on a frenzied attempt to dissect life down to its molecular nuts and bolts, for within the structure of the cell was to be found the heredity mechanism that controlled life."

Dr. Lipton goes on to talk about how scientists have now discovered genes actually control very little. In fact, it is how your genes are EXPRESSED that matters. He says, a new field of study has emerged called epigenetics. Epigenetics is the study of how your environment shapes your gene expression. You are not your genes, but in fact, you are the expression of your genes. Genes can be turned "on" and turned "off". Which genes are expressed (turned "on") will be a result of your environment.

Dr. James Chestnut, a very well known chiropractor, researcher and author of many health and wellness books says, "Your state of health is the genetic expression of your environment. Whatever gene is causing you to have bad health, did not turn its self "on". That gene being turned "on" is the genetic effect of your lifestyle choices."

"The effect of your lifestyle choices bio-accumulate with time. The good news is - your good choices bio-accumulate with time. The bad news is - your bad choices bio-accumulate with time."

When is the best time to start making good healthy choices so you can change your genetic expression? You are absolutely right if you said, "TODAY!"

And the fourth common myth is...

"It is too late for me. "They" said there was nothing I could do".

Please do not fall for this! There is only one time when it truly becomes "too late", and that is right after the last breath has left your body. As Winston Churchill said, "Never, never, never give up!

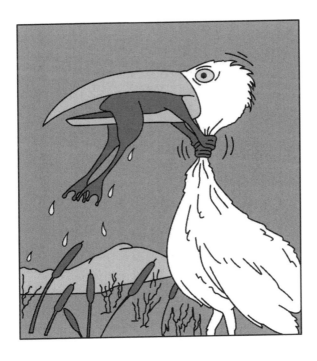

As a chiropractor I sometimes get the patient who has "tried everything". They have been on pain meds, rehab therapy, considered surgery or worse and still haven't got any relief. I have seen these people recover, rebuild and not only survive, but thrive. If you need to make some changes to your health start now!

Trust me; I have been in your shoes before. I would like to share my own personal story with you. My life was completely changed thanks to chiropractic and me making overall lifestyle changes. Now I make it a priority to practice good spinal hygiene, diet, and exercise on a daily bases.

My Story –

When I was a junior in high school, I began to experience strange pains and numbness in my lower back and legs on my way to school every day. My parents were just like most American parents: whenever one of their children had an ache or a pain, they reached for a convenient, over-the-counter pain medicine. For many months this pain continued and became worse. And like most American parents, my mom and dad took me to the doctor, who prescribed pain medication. It was a logical thought: *If the over-the-counter stuff isn't working, Tabor must need something stronger, right?*

Has anyone ever thought that we experience pain for a reason, and until that reason is found and corrected, we will continue to live in pain? I guess not. What a crazy idea.

Well, the prescription pain medication wasn't working either. When the pain and weakness became so bad that I needed help to lift my legs into bed, my parents didn't know what else to do but to take me to the hospital. After a long night and many different, invasive, and very expensive tests, I was sent home with even stronger pain pills and a referral to a neurosurgeon. I'm not sure if someone told my parents about chiropractic care or if they just thought that sounded better than neurosurgery, but making an appointment with a local chiropractor was their next step.

Thank God that was the next step..

The chiropractor took his own x-rays, led us to a room, and proceeded to show us what he found and exactly what he thought was causing my pain. I began receiving adjustments from him every other morning, before school.

My pain was completely gone within three months, and I was a normal 16-year-old once again. You cannot even imagine how wonderful it is to go from being disabled to being well, unless you have been where I was. I have never had that pain again and I am in my 30's now.

That experience proved to me that medicine is not the all-powerful, magic bullet it is portrayed to be. In fact, there is no "magic formula"! Have you ever thought that maybe the magic is within your own body? That "magic" was put there by your Creator. God has given us the power in our own bodies and drug-free remedies found in nature to lead us into lives full of wellness. Natural remedies should not be the alternative. Drugs and surgery should be the alternative! Can you believe we choose what man has created over what God has created every day? That doesn't seem very smart to me.

That is why I have made it a priority to get regular chiropractic care for me and my family and to practice proper spinal hygiene on a daily basis - for the rest of my life!

– Tabor Smith

3

Chiropractic is the Solution

I f you are looking for a real solution to your problem and a great way to make sure your spine stays healthy for a lifetime, you need to discover chiropractic care. Chiropractic has a proven track record. It produces measurable results that last.

Just as dentists correct misaligned teeth with braces, chiropractors correct misaligned spines with chiropractic adjustments (sometimes muscle work and rehab is involved as well).

A misalignment or problem area in the spine is referred to as a vertebral subluxation.

The World Health Organization defines a vertebral subluxation as,

> "A lesion or dysfunction in a joint or motion segment in which alignment, movement integrity and/or physiological function are altered, although contact between joint surfaces remains intact. It is essentially a functional entity, which may influence biomechanical and neural integrity."

Basically a vertebral subluxation is a spinal problem that causes significant health issues in many people and should be corrected as soon as possible and then prevented with proper daily and weekly spinal hygiene procedures. Chiropractors are the only health care professionals that specifically address vertebral subluxations. Subluxations cannot be corrected with drugs or surgery.

Most people have seen before and after pictures of teeth that have been straightened by braces. Correction is a wonderful thing! This dentist has done a great job!...

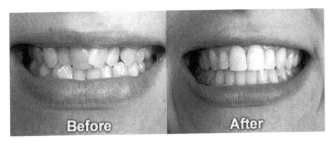

Before and After Braces

Have you ever seen before and after x-rays of people who have had their spine corrected by chiropractor? These chiropractors have done a great job as well!...

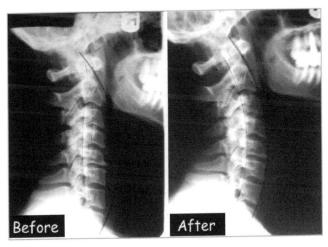

Before   After

(Cervical Spine – side view)

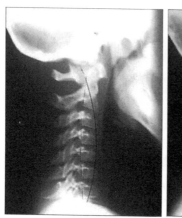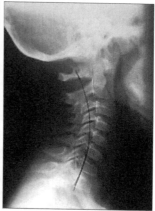

Before   After
(Cervical Spine – side view - 4 yr. old child)

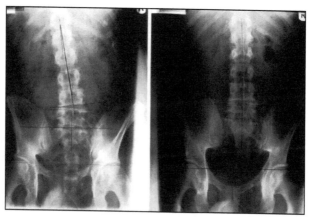

Before   After
(Lumbar Spine – front view)

(Remember from the front the spine should be straight)

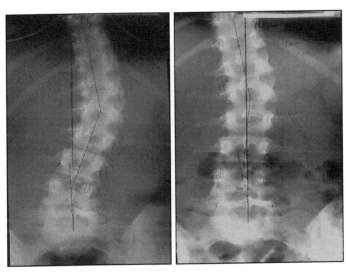

Before   After

(Lumbar Spine – front view)

Those are great examples of chiropractic corrective care. It is a great idea to receive consistent wellness care after your spine has been properly corrected. Although most corrective care plans require multiple visits per week initially, many chiropractors have different recommendations about the frequency of wellness visits.

My family and I get adjusted once a week for wellness and we will for the rest of our lives. Because of that we enjoy great health. I have patients in my office that come once a week, every other week or even once a month for their wellness care. Depending on the condition of your spine your doctor will give you his best recommendations for wellness care.

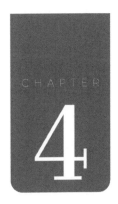

Home Spinal Care Procedures

Spinal hygiene procedures will help you build and maintain the health of your spine by assisting in three different areas. The three areas of spinal health we address here are 1) Spinal Alignment, 2) Spinal Range of Motion, and 3) Spinal Strength and flexibility. These procedures work best when used to maintain the health of the spine rather than restore the health of the spine. As I always say, "Consult your chiropractor before beginning any type of exercise routine."

I understand a lot of the readers of this book are people currently experiencing spinal pain; therefore, I have included Acute Home Spinal Care procedures below. If you are not experiencing spinal pain skip straight to the Daily Home Spinal Care procedures.

If you entered your email address at www.HomeSpinalCare.com you should have been taken to a page with a video. That video will show you some of the Acute Home Spinal Care procedures listed below.

Acute Home Spinal Care Procedures

First, contact your chiropractor and make an appointment as soon as possible. After that, here are some things your chiropractor might suggest.

Ice Therapy

Ice is what I typically recommend for Acute Home Spinal Care. One thing I always say is "When in doubt, use ice." Here are some basic rules you should follow when applying ice therapy:

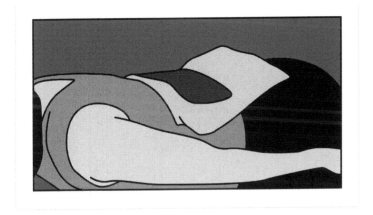

- For acute injuries and swelling, typically within 24-72 hours, use ice therapy only. Apply ice to the central point of pain for 10-15 minutes (NEVER EXCEED 20 MINUTES) at a time. Ice therapy is most commonly applied in the form of an ice pack covered by a dry or moist towel. If you do not have an ice pack, you may substitute a package of frozen vegetables or a frozen bag of un-popped popcorn. This should be done every 2-3 hours and can be applied several times per day. Ice therapy is good for controlling inflammation and swelling which is a major cause of acute pain. (If ice aggravates the condition, stop using immediately and consult your chiropractor.)

Heat Therapy

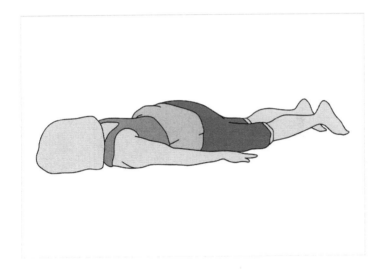

Heat therapy recommendations differ greatly between practitioners. Although heat is usually the first thing people reach for when pain appears. On some occasions heat can cause an increase in inflammation to the affected area. Again, contact your chiropractor and follow his advice. Here are some common directions to follow when applying heat:

- Heat should be used only in more chronic conditions and to help reduce pain and muscle tension. It is best to use moist heat. (Never use the extremely hot or high setting on a heating pad.) Heat should be applied over the area of discomfort for 15-20 minutes per session. (NEVER EXCEED 30 MINUTES.) This should be done every 2-3 hours and can be applied several times per day. (If heat aggravates the condition, stop using immediately and consult your chiropractor)

Contrast Therapy

Perhaps a better use of heat is in what we call contrast therapy. This is the method of rotating ice and heat on the affected area. For people who really enjoy heat more than ice I recommend this method. Here are some directions for applying contrast therapy:

- The combined use of ice and heat is used to increase circulation to an injured area and can be beneficial in reduction of muscle tension. Remember to always start and finish with ice. After the initial application of ice, approximately 5-7 minutes, use a heating pad or hot moist towel for 5-7 minutes, followed again by the use of ice for 5-7 minutes to complete this cycle. You may repeat this cycle for 20-25 minutes per session, and the session may be repeated every 2-3 hours, several times throughout the day. Once again, remember to start and finish with ice.

Getting Comfortable

You may notice with spinal pain (as with any kind of pain) it is hard to get in a comfortable position. It is important not to remain completely immobile as this can sometimes make pains worse and slow healing time (obviously if you suspect serious injury or fracture to the spine, immobilize immediately and call 911 – but, that is not what I'm talking about here).

As far as staying comfortable during back pain here are some directions:

- Rest in a position you find most comfortable. You might try lying on your side with a pillow between your knees. Another position you can try is lying on your back on the floor with a pillow under your knees. Do not stay in one position for too long. Every couple of hours, take a short walk (about 10 to 20 minutes), then find a comfortable position to rest again.

When you and your chiropractor have decided you are ready to move forward with your care you should start the Daily Home Spinal Care procedures below..

Daily Home Spinal Care Procedures

The following Home Spinal Care procedures should be followed daily and consistently just as you brush your teeth. If done correctly and consistently they will help you build and maintain the three areas of spinal health - 1) Spinal Range of Motion, 2) Spinal Alignment, and 3) Spinal Strength and Flexibility. If you entered your email address at www.HomeSpinalCare.com you will also be receiving 3 emails containing videos explaining each Daily Home Spinal Care Procedure below. (If your pain persists, gets worse, or you feel any dizziness with any of the following exercises stop and contact your chiropractor.)

Spinal Range of Motion Stretches

The Why –

A full Spinal range of motion is very important to your spines health. If the joints in the spine are not functioning properly this may alter your spines range of motion. A lack of range of motion has been associated with arthritis and many other spinal diseases.

If you remember from earlier in the book, you have 24 movable segments that make up your spine. These segments are called vertebrae. God could made your spine as one long bone, but he didn't he gave you 24 of them, and he put flexible discs between each one.

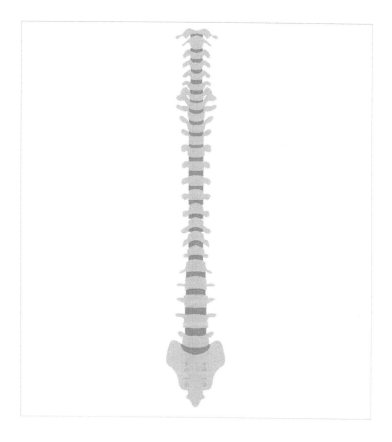

One major benefit of him doing this is the fact you can move! You can twist, turn, bend and stretch all because you have these 24 movable segments called vertebrae.

Dr. Roger Sperry, the 1981 Nobel Prize winner for Brain Research said, "Movement of the joints of the spine is analogous to a windmill generating electricity to run a power plant. Therefore, the more mechanically distorted a person becomes, the less energy there is for healing, metabolism and thinking."

Your spine was made to move! If you want to keep it healthy you have to keep it moving.

<u>The How –</u>

Here are the directions for the Spinal Range of Motion procedure:

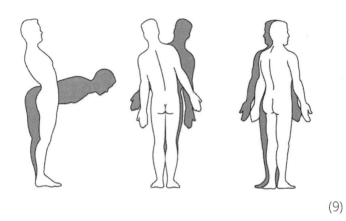

(9)

Lumbar Spine

- Bend forward from a standing position as if you were going to touch your toes. Try to round your spine while keeping the knees bent slightly. Do not bounce or force yourself to go further. Hold this position for 5-10 seconds.

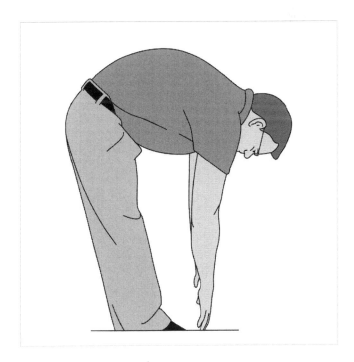

- Bend backward from a standing position while placing hands on your waist and looking up. Hold this position for 5-10 seconds.

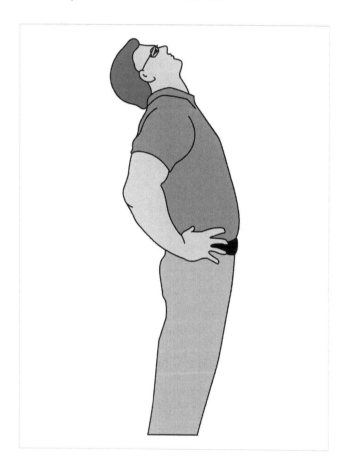

- Place hands straight down to your side and then bend to the left while sliding your left hand down the side of your leg toward your knee. Hold this position for 5-10 seconds.

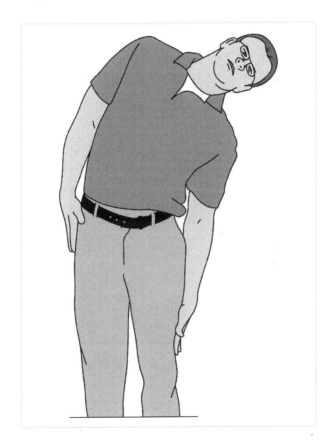

- Place hands straight down to your side and then bend to the right while sliding your right hand down the side of your leg toward your knee. Hold this position for 5-10 seconds.

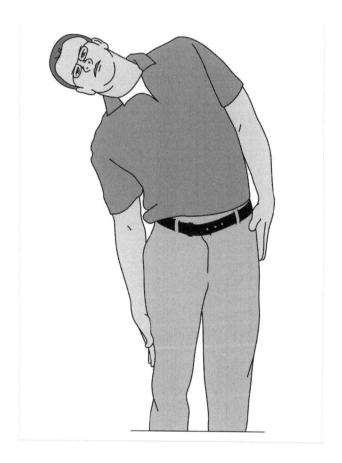

- Place hands together in front of you and twist as far as you can to the left. Do not bounce or try to force yourself to go farther. Hold this position for 5-10 seconds.

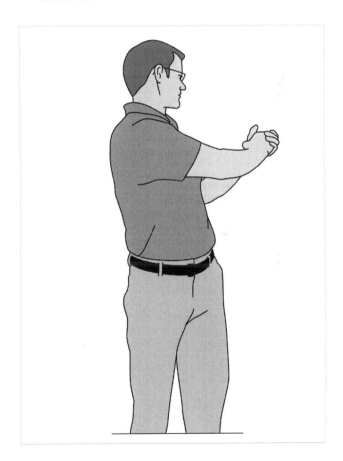

- Place hands together in front of you and twist as far as you can to the right. Do not bounce or try to force yourself to go farther. Hold this position for 5-10 seconds.

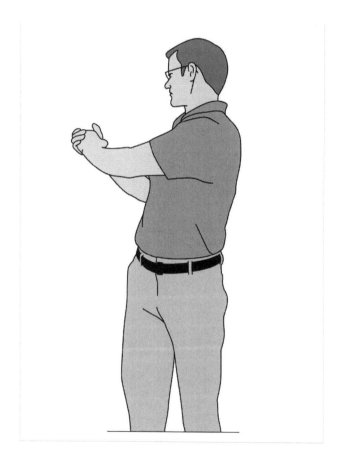

Cervical Spine

- Bend the neck forward as far as you can take your chin to your chest. Hold this position for 5-10 seconds.

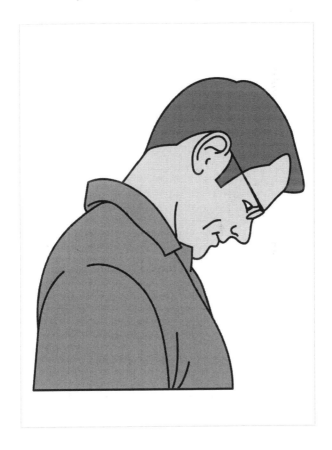

- Bend the neck backward as if you were looking up. (If this motion causes dizziness – stop and contact your chiropractor.). Hold this position for 5-10 seconds..

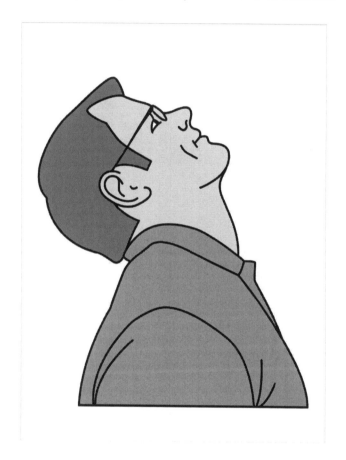

- Bend your neck sideways to the left as if you were going to touch your ear to your shoulder. Hold this position for 5-10 seconds.

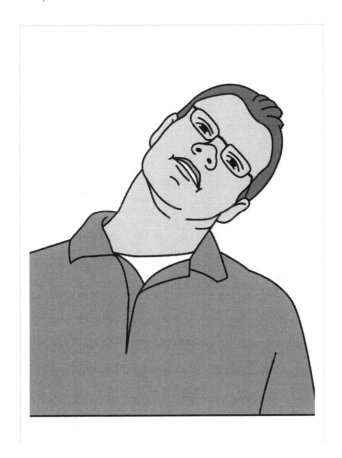

- Bend your neck sideways to the right as if you were going to touch your ear to your shoulder. Hold this position for 5-10 seconds.

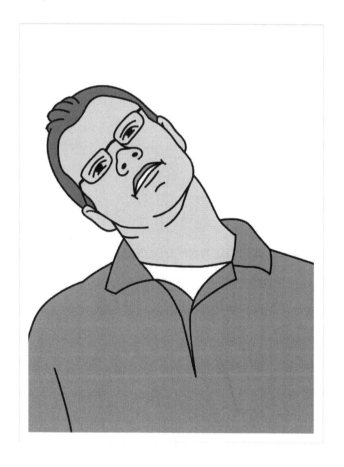

- Turn your neck to the left as far as you can. (If this motion causes dizziness – stop and contact your chiropractor.) Hold this position for 5-10 seconds.

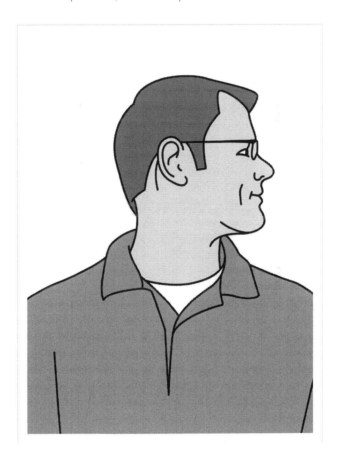

- Turn your neck to the right as far as you can. (If this motion causes dizziness – stop and contact your chiropractor.) Hold this position for 5-10 seconds.

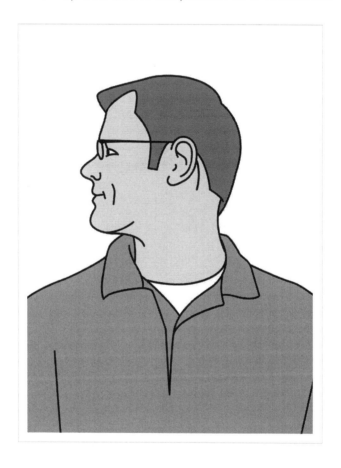

Way to go! You have now taken your spine through its full range of motion. Do this every day to help maintain proper range of motion in your spine. This is also a great exercise to teach your children so they can grow up practicing proper spinal hygiene.

Postural Strengthening Exercises

The Why -

It is well known that core and postural muscles provide spinal stability. So it goes without saying, we need to keep these muscles active and strong. They say it takes 90 days to develop permanent muscle change. This means it is very important that you are consistent with your daily spinal care procedures.

Three inches of forward head poster can cause the head to feel like it weighs up to 42 pounds! Just think of the pressure that puts on the vertebrae and the spinal cord. By strengthening postural muscles we can help take some unnecessary pressure off the spine.

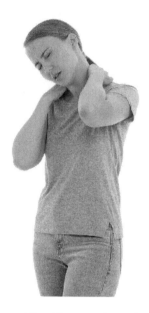

"For every inch of Forward Head Posture, it can increase the weight of the head on the spine by an additional 10 pounds."

(From Kapandji, Physiology of Joints, Vol. 3)

Even the Mayo Clinic said, (Nov. 3rd, 2000) "Anterior Head Syndrome leads to long term muscle strain, disc herniations, arthritis and pinched nerves."

By strengthening core and postural muscles in both the neck and back we can decrease stress on the spine, therefore, maintaining the health of our nervous system.

<u>The how –</u>

Here are the directions for the Postural Strengthening procedures:

Cervical Postural Muscles

....

- Take an elastic band, put it around the back of your head and hold the ends straight out in front of you with both hands equal distance from your head. (Make sure to inspect your band for tears each time and hold on tightly to the ends of the band so that it does not release unexpectedly and "pop" you in the face.)

- Extend your elbows and hold tension on the band while looking straight a head and tucking the chin back. It is very important to keep proper technique everytime you do this exercise.

- Hold the tension on the band for 10 seconds then release and rest for 10 seconds. Repeat this 3 times.

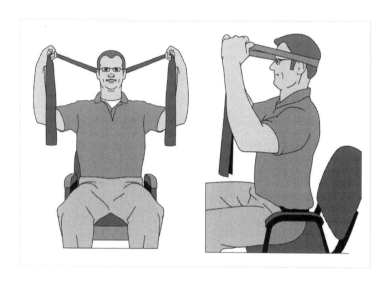

Lumbar/Core Muscles

- Place your exercise disc in the seat of your chair. (It is recommended to use a chair that has arms so that you can hold the arms if you need to balance.) I like to put a little more air in my exercise disc, but a flat disc will work just fine.

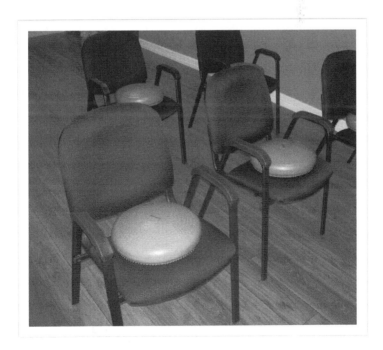

- You will do 4 exercises on your exercise disc. The first exercise you do while sitting on your exercise disc is bending forward and back. ↕ (Put a C in your spine forward and then a C in your spine backward.) Bend forward and back 10 times.

- The second exercise you do while sitting on your exercise disc is bending side to side. ↔ (Put a C in your spine to the left and then put a C in your spine to the right.) Bend side to side 10 times

- The third exercise you do while sitting on your exercise disc is rotation to the left. ↻ (Rotate your waste around in circles as if you were using a hula hoop.) Rotate to the left 10 times.

- The fourth exercise you do while sitting on your exercise disc is rotation to the right. ↺ (Rotate your waste around in circles as if you were using a hula hoop.) Rotate to the right 10 times.

-

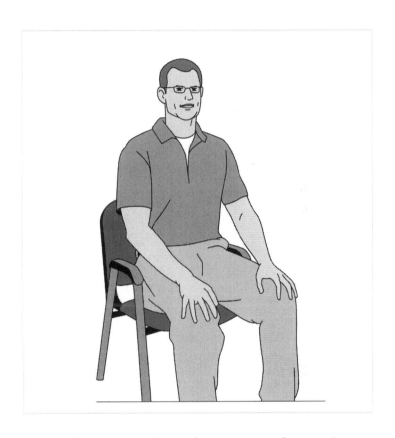

- The exercise disc is also a great tool to use in your office chair (or any chair you use a lot) as you sit during the day. It will help to activate core muscles and balance as you work.

Spinal Molding

The Why -

To understand what Spinal Molding is and why it is so important you must first understand a couple very interesting things about the discs of the spine (Discs are the padding between each vertebrae). According to Dr. Dennis Woggon, founder of CLEAR INSTITUTE for scoliosis correction, the inside of the disc contains a gel-like material that can go from a hydrogel (firm) state to a hydrosol (fluid) state when we exercise our spine. In other words, motion loosens the gel and a lack of motion will allow the gel to harden.

Another very interesting fact about the spine is that after the age of puberty the spinal discs become avascular (having no blood supply). Motion of the spine becomes the only way for the disc to stay healthy.

How does motion of the spine keep discs healthy you ask? By a process known as imbibition, the "pumping" or movement of the spine when exercising forces nutrients in and waste material out of the spinal disc. That is one reason why arthritis can ensue when a spinal segment is fixated (no longer moving properly). (3)

Spinal Molding allows us to take advantage of these spinal properties. We start with an exercise that "pumps" the disc and provides nutrients (imbibition). It also loosens the inter-gel material so we can mold the proper curves into the spine by lying on foam rolls and allowing the inter-gel material to harden.

The How -

Here are directions for the Spinal Molding procedure:

- Sit on the edge of a bed or chair. Make sure you are sitting up very straight and looking slightly upward. Raise shoulders forward to 90 degrees and bend elbows inward to 90 degrees so the knuckles of your hands are touching. You then twist back and forth 15-25 times. (IF you have trouble with dizziness try looking up more, twisting slower, or if dizziness persists or pain becomes worse stop the exercise and contact your chiropractor.)

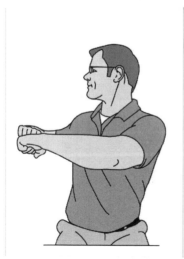 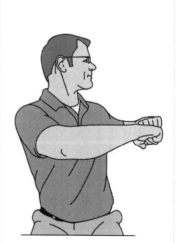

- After you finish the spinal twist exercise lay on your back. Take two foam rolls, lay one under the curve of your neck (right above the shoulders) and the other under the curve of your low back. Lay on these rolls for 15-20 minutes to al-low the spinal discs to return to a hydro-gel state (firm). This will help to mold the natural curves into the spine, maintaining proper alignment, relieving muscle tension and helping to take pressure off of the nerves.

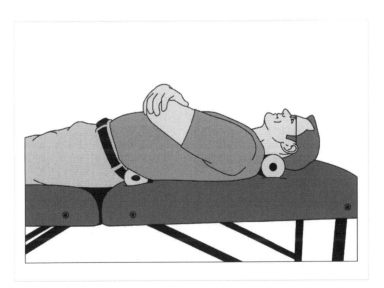

It is also very beneficial to sleep on a cervical sleep aid from time to time. I try to fall asleep on mine every night. Usually I wake up in the middle of the night sometime, toss it aside, and grab my pillow, but even then, that is hours of spinal molding that are being done every night. I highly recommend it.

- Lie on your back in bed and take a soft foam roll, place it under the curve of your neck (right above the shoulders just as you do for the spinal molding exercise above). Try to fall asleep while laying on your back using only the cervical sleep aid (soft foam roll) as your pillow. If you cannot fall asleep just lay on it for 15-20 minutes and take it out. (Stop if you feel pain or dizziness and contact your chiropractor)

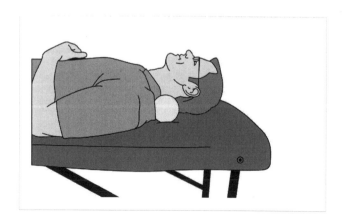

Summary

You can do each of these exercises 1-2 times per day (along with regular chiropractic visits) they will help keep your spine healthy and well. Even if you just do a couple of them several times a week that is better than most people, who do nothing at all and expect their spine to stay in good shape. When it comes to the spine the old saying is true, "If you don't move it, you loose it."

 When you have an injury or a flare up (call you chiropractor and then) use the Acute Home Spinal Care Procedures you learned.

 As you go through your day stop and do the Spinal Range of Motion Stretches you learned.

 Take your exercise disk to the office and put it in the chair you sit in all day.

 Try to fit your elastic band neck exercises in to your day as well.

 Before you go to sleep at night do the spinal molding exercise.

I know that sounds like a lot, but if you get into a habit of practicing proper spinal hygiene you will not only feel better and have a healthier spine, but you will be able to enjoy life to the fullest!

If you have found this book helpful please
tell a friend about it so they can understand
how to take care of their spine also!

(Copy and Paste the link below – Then email it to your friends!)

www.HomeSpinalCare.com

Bibliography

1) "Answers.com - What Does the Nervous System Do for You." WikiAnswers - The Q&A Wiki. Answers.com. Web. 13 May 2011. http://wiki.answers.com/Q/What_does_the_nervous_system_do_for_you

2) "What Is Chiropractic?" ACAToday.org. American Chiropractic Association. Web. 13 May 2011 http://www.acatoday.org/level2_css.cfm?T1ID=13&T2ID=61.

3) H.F. Farfan in Managing Low Back Pain by Kirkaldy-Willis, Churchill Livingstone (1983) p.19

Made in the USA
Columbia, SC
02 September 2022

66400928R00046